CONGRATULATIONS ON YOUR DECISION TO GET HEALTHY!

SOUPS & SALADS

COOKBOOK XII

A guide to a *new eating plan* that is not a "DIET", created based on personal experience to help you *finally* achieve your weight loss and health goals.

ALSO BY KYLA LATRICE, MBA

"New Me, New You! (How I Overcame Obesity)"

"The 7 Day Smoothie Detox"

"The 21 Day Slushie & Juice Fast"

"The 21 Day Salad Fast"

"Eat Well and Stay Thin (Living a Healthy You)"

"21 Days to a New Healthy You! Hearty Vegan & Vegetarian
Slow Cooker Recipes"

"Twenty-One Healthy Ice Pop Snack Recipes"

"21 Days of Everyday Healthy Snack Recipes"

"All Natural Soups & Stews"

"A Collection of My Favorite Health Recipes"

"A New You! Workout Workbook"

SOUPS & SALADS

A 21 DAY SOUPS & SALADS GUIDE TO RESET YOUR HEALTH, MIND, BODY, METABOLISM AND *"LIFE"*

KYLA LATRICE, MBA

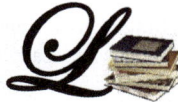

Lady Mirage Publications, Inc.

New York   Memphis   Los Angeles   London   Cape Town   Toronto
Atlanta   Singapore   Japan

Published by:
Lady Mirage Publications, Inc.
3724 Goodman Rd W, Unit 575
Horn Lake, MS 38637
www.LadyMirageAgency.com

Manufactured in the United States of America
First Edition: April 2015

Lady Mirage Publications, Inc. is an imprint and subsidiary
of Lady Mirage Global. The Lady Mirage Publications, Inc. name
and logo are trademarks of Lady Mirage Global.

Authors within the Lady Mirage Global (under Lady Mirage Agency,
Inc.), Lady Mirage Publications and Lady Mirage Literary Agency
speakers division provides a wide range of authors for speaking
engagements. To find out more information, go to
www.LadyMirageAgency.com
Cover photo provided by lkunl at FreeDigitalPhotos.net
The publisher is not responsible for websites (or their content) that
are not owned by the publisher.

Library of Congress Cataloging-in-Publication Data:
eISBN: 978-1-31-194831-1; Print ISBN: 978-0-9975371-9-2
Tennin, Kyla Latrice.
Soups & Salads
Pages cm; copyrighted materials.
1.   Health-Nutrition-Diet-Fitness. 2. Cooking. 3. Fitness.
Library of Congress Catalog Card Number: 2016907242

Print Book Edition, License Note

Also Note

In this book, Ms. Latrice begins by explaining a *fast* that she has created, tested and tried, which contributed to her weight loss, weight management and healthy eating lifestyle journey.
She has also written this book due to there being so many books, health, weight-loss and "diet" programs currently on the global market. The programs and books she has seen and reviewed are too long, too thick, have too much information and many times, are difficult for people to read. This book was written to *simplify and shorten* how to lose weight and maintain your health, for life. It is based on personal experience and is still done today. It's an effective solution.

Soups & Salads

Table of Contents

SOUPS & SALADS RECIPES..**40**

Day 1: Good Old-Fashioned Vegetarian Soup..........42

        Day 2: Garlic Chicken Salad……...................……44

Day 3: Cabbage & Barley Soup...........................46

        Day 4: Quinoa Salad with Pears Salad...............48

Day 5: Tomato Basil Soup…................................50

        Day 6: Avocado Dill Salad...........................……52

Day 7: Radishes & Green Onion Soup....................54

        Day 8: Pineapple Dill Remix..........................56

Day 9: Spinach & Wild Mushrooms Soup…....………58

        Day 10: Salmon Carrot Lime Salad...........………60

Day 11: All Natural Grains Soup…...........……….62

        Day 12: Quinoa Pesto Salad….........................64

Day 13: White Bean & Rosemary Soup..................66

        Day 14: Summer Kiwi Salad.....................……68

Day 15: Beats & Celery Soup……...................…..70

        Day 16: Tilapia Fajita Salad…...……….....……...72

Day 17: Sun Dried Tomato & Avocado Soup...........74

        Day 18: Cucumber Feta Salad with Balsamic.......76

Day 19: Asparagus Soup…................……...…....78

        Day 20: Shrimp Avocado Salad...……….....……82

Day 21: Broccoli Soup…...........................…….80

INDEX...……...**84**

        Soups & Salad Recipes………...…………84

DEDICATION

This cookbook is dedicated to men and women around the
world that have dealt with or are beginning to deal with food
addiction, obesity and/or declining health.

I also dedicate this book to those whom have been "Mirage's"
in life; overlooked, betrayed, not good enough, slandered,
mistreated, misunderstood, misrepresented and even treated
unfairly because of their weight or how they looked on the
outside to others, when in fact, on the *inside* there's greater.

This new cookbook is also dedicated to men and women
around the world that want to
shift from being ordinary to extraordinary and accomplishing
what others said you would never be able to do again or never
be able to do at all.

Here's to the New You!

ACKNOWLEDGMENTS

I want to *say thank you* to anyone whom has ever betrayed,
rejected, mistreated, teased, and misused
or looked down upon me. You helped me become GREATER
and launched me into my destiny.

Whenever someone throws bricks at you, use them to *"build"*.
Build something greater; even your mansion.

And whenever you face opposition, "know" that it is actually
an opportunity; a set-back for a set-up to secure the victory,
rejection for rewards, pain for gain, lack for prosperity to
leave a legacy, misery for miracles and put downs for
promotion.

IT'S YOUR TIME...*to bounce back!*

Let's Get Healthy!

AUTHOR'S NOTE

AFFIDAVIT

All content written herein is of opinion, from personal
experience and of suggestion. Individual salad fast and new
eating plan results may vary from person to person and no
results are guaranteed.

You must put forth effort and do the work necessary to take
charge of changing your life and *losing weight*. I did and so
can you.

You can also utilize this cookbook if you have already met
your weight loss goals and just want to stay healthy with
recipes that will keep your metabolism in check and body
running smoothly.

Be sure to wash all fruits, vegetables, foods, etc. thoroughly
before beginning any new
eating or meal plan.

ALL RIGHTS RESERVED

"ON-THE-GO"

This cookbook *(and all of my cookbooks,*
books, workbook and manuals) can be read and applied in
airports, on trains, at work on your lunch break,
in grocery stores while shopping for and planning your
weekly meals, at bookstore cafes,
at restaurants *(for quick decision making; to remember your*
health and/or weight loss goals) and even in shopping malls.

In addition, *this book can be brought to*
fast food restaurants (to pull up and look through to remember
your goals before ordering), at the park (before a jog or
potluck), during your hotel stays,
on vacations and at airport food counters when ordering your
meals and drinks *(so you remember your goals and what to*
eat and drink).

This cookbook has been made available
on mobile devices via Adobe Digital Editions and DRM
(Digital Rights Management).

WORLD STATISTICS

Obesity and Childhood Obesity
Centers for Disease Control and Prevention
http://www.cdc.gov/obesity/data/adult.html
http://www.cdc.gov/nchs/fastats/obesity-overweight.htm

Harvard School of Public Health
http://www.hsph.harvard.edu/obesity-prevention-
source/obesity-trends/

World Health Organization
http://www.who.int/topics/obesity/en/

Stroke Awareness and Prevention
http://www.cdc.gov/stroke/facts.htm

Diabetes Awareness and Prevention
Centers for Disease Control and Prevention
http://www.cdc.gov/diabetes/data/statistics/2014statisticsrepor
t.html

American Diabetes Association
http://www.diabetes.org/diabetes-basics/statistics/

"FASTING"

WHAT IS FASTING?

➢ Fasting is abstaining from PLEASURABLE foods for a certain amount of time to FOCUS on things that are more important than pleasurable foods to get to the root of what is causing your poor health, obesity, relationships and quality of life.

➢ It is not a hunger strike.

➢ You're able to see into your life better and rid it of the bad when you pull away from portion after portion at the dinner table, lunch buffet after buffet with friends and co-workers, nightly binge eating and drinking (whether alcohol, sodas, sugary drinks and the like) and dessert or movie nights on the sofa with a large pizza box and donuts.

➢ Fasting helps you pinpoint where you overdo things (overindulge), gets you back on track and teaches you how to eat, "in moderation" (balance), for your health and for a better life.

➢ Your body may not like eating healthy for the first few days (especially if you have never fasted before), but it will adjust.

REASONS FOR FASTING:

➢ It produces a physical discipline (especially for how, when, where and *what* you eat).

➢ It rids the body of toxins (just like exercise does when you sweat); cleansing your body and digestive tracts, improving your health and weight.

Note: If you are on medication, consult your physician before any *fast*.

BENEFITS OF FASTING:
- It strengthens *you* and your body.

- Fasting brings joy, happiness and *energy* to your life; and fruits, vegetables, oils, etc. are quite inexpensive. Make a list and shop for your ingredients before you begin.

- You become very aware of *what* and *how much* you eat. You also begin to pay more attention to when and where you always eat/drink and what leads you to OVEREATING.

- Fasting brings humility, revelation and an overall healthy lifestyle (mind, emotions, intellect, etc.).

TYPICAL TYPES OF FASTS:
Sometimes people fast the following from their lives:
- Television (even the internet, social media or video games) for one day, three days or even one week, television during certain hours of the day (to break a cycle of watching certain shows they may be addicted to (like food) that aren't good for them.
        ....or
- To break a cycle of "certain foods" they may eat while watching certain television shows.

- Fasting to abstain from all pleasurable foods and red meats, eating only fruits, vegetables, clear soups, cereals (no white sugar), water, diluted fruit juices (100% juices only) and/or grains.

- Some people even fast people (bad acquaintances, friendships or relationships), leading eventually to moving away from those person's completely, for a better life and health. Your health is your life.

➤ Many people fast for 24 hours, three days, seven days, 14 days, 21 days or longer. My success and learning my body as well as other persons bodies (whom have fasted when I have fasted) has come from "closely monitoring" how the body reacts to each of these fasts (particularly "21 days") and I've noticed some things and have sculpted recipes to help others find that tremendous success in many areas of their lives as well.

➤ Fasts should always be broken slowly, especially if you have been on an "extended fast" (a fast for more than 30 days, a salad only fast, a smoothie only fast or even a clear soup only fast).

➤ Gradually get back into "regular food", until you can completely commit to "healthy food" (and a regular healthy lifestyle); such as having juices for a couple of days, then fruits, vegetables, grains and adding meats back into your diet last, if applicable.

➤ Typically, people have six meals per day (three main meals (breakfast, lunch and dinner) and three snacks). For each of my Fasts or Recipes, you determine how many meals. Don't worry, fruits and vegetables do not cause obesity, they prevent it. Yet, always watch your portion sizes, in general, and with soups, stews and anything that has meat included. Never eat meat in excess.

➤ You can even choose to eat one meal per day for 21 days (there are enough recipes listed in this book), a snack, have 5-8 bottles of water and be sure to get a nap in and some exercise during the week. As you advance you can mix your salad fast with a smoothie fast and detox fast by doing one of the fasts, each per week, for 21 days, etc.

THE *"SALAD FAST"* BIRTH

Kyla Latrice is a native of Marks, MS and enjoys food and traveling. Being from a small town and a country gal, she set her goals high. Graduating from a private institution with a Bachelor of Arts Degree (BA) *(women's studies and health background; pre-medicine)* and a Master's Degree (MBA) in Business Administration with **Executive Education at Harvard and Stanford** along with several certifications and nearly 50-80 self-study coursework in legal, intellectual property and self-help, she has become one of the leading entrepreneurs of her time.

Currently Ms. Latrice is finishing up her Doctoral Honorary Degree *(Doctor of Management in Organizational Leadership)* and continues to serve on Board of Directors throughout the world for various causes; still relating to her life's purpose and corporations work. Ms. Latrice travels extensively for speaking engagements in the areas of health, wellness, obesity, poverty, domestic violence, branding, image, leadership, mentoring, business, entrepreneurship and the like.

To date, Ms. Latrice has mentored with over 20 plus organizations *(from elementary to senior citizen)*, helping others overcome issues she has faced.

With her first *corporate* job opportunity being at a "Health Food Restaurant" *(when she was age 15 or 16)* to work as a deli attendant at the deli bar, hostess *(when others were out for the day)* and bakery attendant as well as a chef in the *salad bar*.

Her main role was to attend to the deli, to prepare healthy pasta salads, healthy sandwiches, healthy shakes, healthy sundaes and *healthy smoothies*. However, Ms. Latrice was blessed with the opportunity to be called upon whenever management needed her help in the other areas as well, **to continue learning**. This gave Ms. Latrice very valuable experience and a "look" into health and business ownership, a bit deeper, which still remains with her today.

THE *"SALAD FAST"* BIRTH

KYLA LATRICE
BEFORE
21 DAY SALAD FASTS

Ms. Latrice's *(on the left in the photo)*
Corporations are inclusive of health restaurants, retail
stores, property and land as well as product development
organizations along with nonprofit foundations to care for
the displaced, homeless.

Further, Ms. Latrice's love for food turned into
obesity when her life took a turn in the early 2000's during
domestic violence, sinful relationships, bad friendships and
emotional binge eating; then again in the 2000's with
another domestic violence relationship, obesity slander
from family members, mental and spiritual abuse, abortion,
home foreclosure, vehicle repossession and much *more*,
which all have an effect on health, but she made sure her
Corporations still stood; to help others.

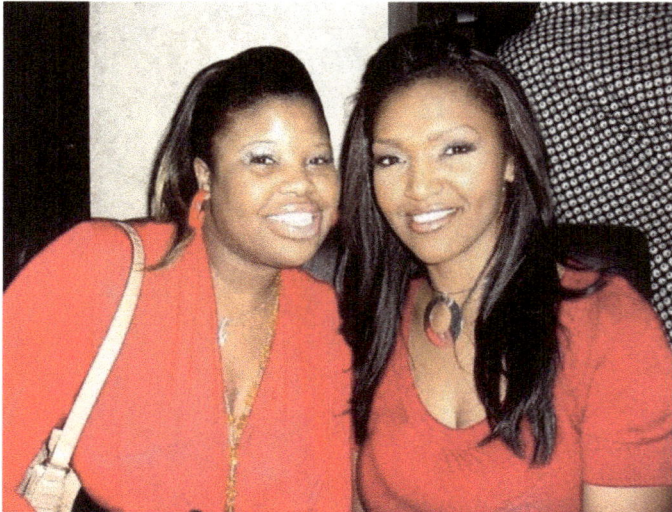

THE *"SALAD FAST"* BIRTH

KYLA LATRICE
"IN THE MIDDLE"
AFTER GAINING WEIGHT BACK FOR A SECOND TIME
21 DAY SALAD FASTS

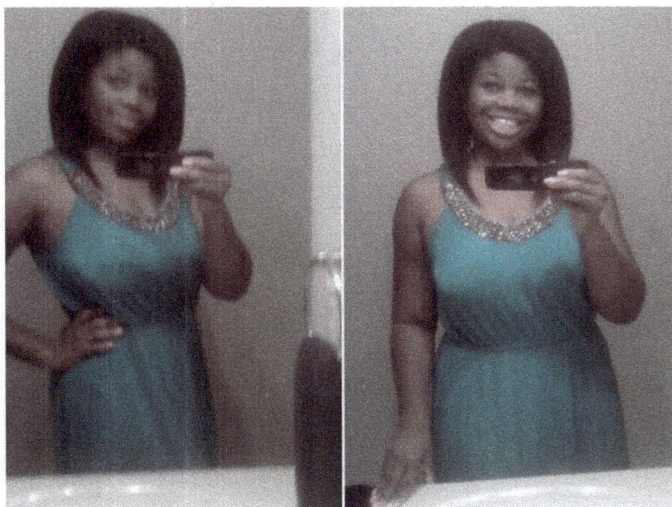

THE *"SALAD FAST"* BIRTH

KYLA LATRICE
AFTER
21 DAY SALAD FASTS

THE FINALE

Many factors can contribute to obesity, such as abuse *(mental, spiritual, physical, sexual)*, poor eating habits, environment, bad friendships as well as sin. Personally, I, myself, was never taught how to eat, I did not know what to eat *(that was truly healthy for me)* and I did not know how to deal with life's problems.

Nevertheless, how can someone teach you what they don't know? My first encounter with obesity was when I was a model and went from a size 0 to a size 20/22, **weighing close to 300 pounds** *(then I lost nearly 115 pounds after prayer and seeking a remedy)*.

The second encounter was when I gained some of the first encounters weight back and went from a size 14/16 to a size 4/6 and fitting a 7/8 in jeans, losing 68 pounds. Today, I am going to share my secrets to success with you *(the birth of the "21 Day Salad Fast")* and how I made it out over the years ***and*** kept the weight off. Let's get started and healthy, for life!

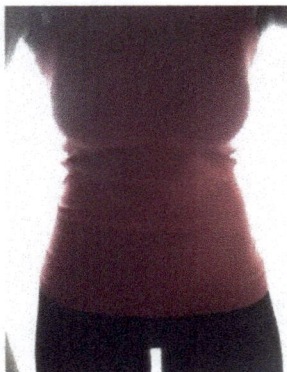

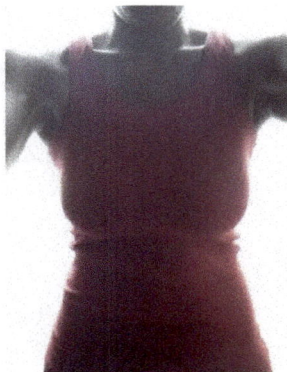

GETTING HEALTHY
LIFESTYLE CHANGE

Prepare to lose weight on the "Salad Fast" (this is not a "diet", this is an "eating plan" to reprogram your mind, body and metabolism about how to eat (portion control) and regarding what foods you should and should not be eating). It is designed to help you become healthier. Before starting this fast and any of my eating *plans ("The 21 Day Smoothie Fast" and "The 21 Day Salad Fast" as well as "Soups and Stews"),* allow yourself "one week" to prepare for the fast and eating plan by removing the following from your life:

➢ Negative relationships and friendships; they block you from doing well in life and succeeding, when people begin to see you doing well, they tend to not like it. Choose friendships and associations wisely. Be creative.

➢ Bad acquaintances; they will eventually want what you have and will cause betrayal to take place in your life through a "set-up" to sabotage all of your hard work. Always keep moving forward.

➢ Remove the following (slowly) from your daily meals (eating habits) because they contribute to weight gain (some quicker than others): soda, breads, pastas, candy bars and the like and eating second, third and fourth portions of your food. You only need one portion. Don't eat the rest!

➢ Replace all sodas with diet soda until you can cut soda out of your daily meal plan completely; only drink soda if absolutely necessary *(a lemon-lime beverage)* because there is nothing else to drink. For example, while traveling.

➢ Remove all "junk food" (cakes, pies, chips, all kinds of desserts and the like) from your kitchen.

➤ For breads, certain kinds make the weight gain skyrocket; be careful about pizza. Pasta should be limited just like soda, having it only if absolutely necessary, but once every 2-4 months is okay, just like donuts, to stay *balanced* and give your body a break from always eating healthy.

➤ Again, you only need one portion of food, per meal, work on this and you'll see results quicker.

➤ Increase your water intake to 5-8 bottled waters a day; bring a bottle with you everywhere you go so you'll be forced to drink it *(instead of something else)* and will program your body to like it *(whether you like it frozen, warm or cold)*.

➤ When you're out to eating with others, begin selecting items from menus that help *(not hinder)* your **new eating plan**, for example, order a "grilled chicken wrap with a side salad and small water" instead of a double cheeseburger, french fries and large soda. Never super-size, it wastes your results and time spent on improving your health.

➤ If you have not already, purchase my books: *"The 21 Day Smoothie Fast"* and *"The 7 Day Detox"* to begin, to continue your weight loss and new you.

➤ And again, remember, commit to single portion eating, eating smaller portions (always have more vegetables on your plate than poultry/ meat), and increase your water intake *(remember to use the restroom)*. Let's begin.

GETTING HEALTHY
SET GOALS

Feel free to purchase my "A New Healthy You Workout Workbook" *(to go with your **new eating plan** and my "fasts" cookbooks* or a composition notebook from any retailer to make your own journal to measure the following (even if you need to do so at your primary care physician's office, a free clinic or go to a free health assessment machine in a retail store location that has one):

Record a written record of each:

> ➢ Your Cholesterol Level.
> ➢ Blood Pressure and Vision Check.
> ➢ Your actual Height Weight, Height, Bust/Chest and Hips size (write down your goals of where you want to be in the next week, three months, six months and year).
> ➢ Record your weight, chest/bust, hips and waist size every Saturday morning at 7am.
> ➢ Stroll through a department store and notate clothing (or take a camera phone photo) you plan on fitting into someday and notate your current sizes and then return in three months to see how you're fairing up towards your goals.
> ➢ Pick up my *"A New Healthy You Workout Workbook"* or list in your journal, your reasons for losing weight, changing your life and changing your eating habits.

> Your BMI (Body Mass Index) and where you are versus where you're supposed to be for your height, weight, age and gender.
> Bottles of "cold water" listed in the recipes section of this book are in reference to drinking 4-5 bottles of 16 fl oz bottles of water, which is equivalent to 8-10 glasses of water per day.
> Water is vital for living and for being healthy.
> The amount of water within the human body is typically 50-65% water and in infants, 78%.
> Water assists your body with digesting food and getting nutrients from the foods you have eaten to your blood, brain and other parts of your body, in order to function; emptying the body of waste and toxins, helps deliver oxygen to the body, helps prevent constipation and even regulates body temperature (in your cells, organs and tissues).

A (BMI) Chart is below for your convenience.

BMI	<(less than) 18.5	=	Underweight
BMI	18.5-24.9	=	Normal Weight
BMI	25-29.9	=	Overweight
BMI	>(more than) 30	=	Obese

GETTING HEALTHY
WHILE TRAVELING

If you'll be traveling by airplane, helicopter or private jet (smile):

➢ Research where you will be eating ahead of time (food choices, ingredients and prices).
➢ Bring bottled water.
➢ Resist vending machines and relying of fast food at your final destination.
➢ Bring your own snacks (trail mix, cashews, a banana, apple slices, peanuts) and
➢ Workout for free in your hotel room, taking the stairs instead of elevators and walking at the Mall.

If traveling by car:

➢ Pack your own cooler with ice for your bottled waters, fruits and raw vegetables.
➢ Consider bringing a bag of oranges & any other food that can be eaten warm or cold on the road.

If you'll be traveling by bus, train, or other means:

➢ Research where you will be eating ahead of time (food choices, ingredients and prices).
➢ Bring bottled water.
➢ Bring your own snacks (trail mix, cashews, a banana, apple slices, peanuts for the long trip) and
➢ Bring something to read or play, to keep your mind off of food and *fictious* hunger.
➢ At your destination, stand more than you sit (to keep your body moving) and since you have been sitting during traveling for your trip.

GREEN BEANS

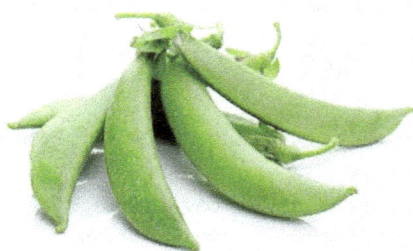

GETTING HEALTHY
YOUR NEW WORKOUT PLAN

During my both times of being obese, I never worked out at a gym nor went outside of my home to run *(weighing in at 278 pounds and trying to start my "new me" as a jogger was terrible on my knees)* to lose weight, I did it all at home, on the floor, in a compact room, near a closet. I suggest you begin a "workout regime" by doing simple workouts, such as crunches, stretching, leg lifts and a few push-ups.

Everyone cannot do cardio in the gym (paid membership prices or because of lack of transportation), running outside or bouncing around in-doors for 1-3 hours like actors and actresses on television, whom are likely being *paid monetary* compensation or by other means to film the infomercial.

Remain constant and do this 3-4 times a week, for 15-35 minutes each day. On your workout OFF days, do 100 crunches before going to bed. Consider purchasing my "Workout Workbook" to keep up with your Fitness Plan. In addition, you burn calories when you sleep, by drinking water, by exercising (which helps you live longer as well) and by **movement** (whether your arms, legs, looking out of a window, etc.).

Furthermore, water helps break down food and helps food digest. Your can also do a "mental workout" by cutting out negative people, places and things from your life.

You'll find that you have more peace in your brain and life, when you replace them with reading inspirational books, movies, community work and exercise or things you love, such as knitting, a ball game, taking a site seeing road trip (alone) every now and then or mentoring someone.

Notes

_____
_____
_____
_____
_____
_____
_____
_____
_____
_____
_____
_____
_____
_____
_____
_____
_____
_____
_____
_____
_____
_____
_____
_____
_____

THE SIX MONTH RULE
GIVE IT *"TIME"*

THE SIX-MONTH RULE

On a 21-Day Salad Fast, weight [pounds] have been known to drop quickly for many people. However, the goal here is to also keep the weight off. Stay focused and be committed to at least six-months of "health work".

Remember to journal your progress.

There's something about when you write things down, they get *ACCOMPLISHED!* Also give yourself a total of six-months to work on your "New You" simply because you may lose inches first and not weight, until your weight catches up with your inches (this is what took place with me; loosing 10-12 pounds per month).

Inches first then one day the weight just fell off. And for others, sometimes weight first, then inches.

GO BACK TO THE DEPARTMENT STORE

Revisit those same department stores that you went to on the first week of your new lifestyle change, try on new clothing sizes to see where you are with your goals.

I suggest that you "mentally shop" for a new suit, a dinner dress, clothing for you next vacation (Hawaii maybe), your first pair of skinny jeans or baseball gear to wear to a game; all after you have reached your goals; to *CELEBRATE!*

"SOUPS & SALADS"
RECIPES

WEEK 1
ARUGULA WEEK

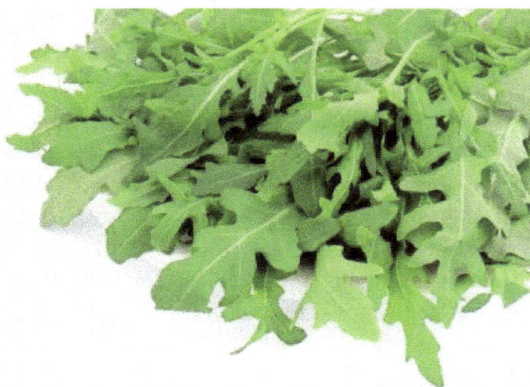

Photo Credit: Apolonia
FREEDIGITALPHOTOS.NET

WEEK 1, DAY 1
(GOOD OLD-FASHIONED VEGETARIAN SOUP)

Day 1 of Week 1: Typically makes 4-6 servings and lasts a few days, but utilize a "Small" Boiler Pot or "Small Sized Crock-Pot" (for best results) for smaller portions to watch your weight, prevent over-eating and watch your sodium (salt) intake.

Main Ingredients:
Into a Small Boiler Pot
Certified 100% Organic (home grown is best) Vegetables

Add 1 cup of diced onion, Add 1 cup of diced green bell pepper, Add 1 cup of diced red bell pepper, Add 1 cup of corn, Add 1 cup of diced parsley, Add 1 cup of diced roma tomatoes (both yellow and red), Add 1 cup of diced celery, Add a dash of salt, Add 1/2 teaspoon of ground red pepper, Add a dash of pepper, Add 1 diced garlic clove, Add 1/2 teaspoon of thyme, Add 2 teaspoons of certified 100% organic extra-virgin olive oil, Add 4-5 cups of (purified) water (regular cold tap water is fine as well), Bring to a boil

Cook for a few hours
Cook until thoroughly heated and boiled
Serve immediately, after cooling (5-10 minutes)

Additional Notes: if desired:
Add 1 cup of any (diced) 100% certified organic, farm raised, grass fed "baked" lemon-pepper and Greek seasoned meat

Weight Loss Tip: Drink 4-5 bottles of cold water today.

LEMONS

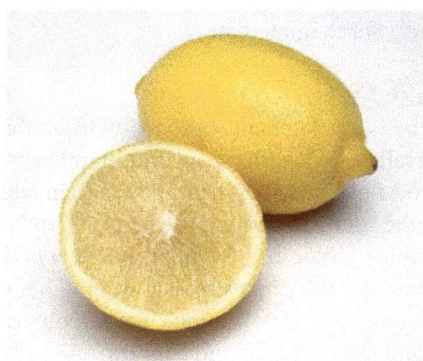

Photo Credit: Suat Eman
FREEDIGITALPHOTOS.NET

WEEK 1, DAY 2
(GARLIC CHICKEN)

Day 2 of Week 1: Garlic, Extra-Virgin Olive Oil, Fresh Lemon Juice, Shredded Skinless Boneless Rotisserie Chicken Breast, Green Onions

Add 1/2 teaspoon of minced garlic into a large salad bowl, Add 3 tablespoons of extra-virgin olive oil, Add 1/2 of a lemon's squeezed juice, Add 1 cup of shredded skinless boneless rotisserie chicken breast, 1/2 cup of diced green onions, Mix salad with large serving spoon until evenly mixed, Place on a bed of baby arugula on a dinner plate or in a to go container, Serve immediately

Health Notes:

Garlic – Garlic is an excellent source of nutrient that promotes overall body health. It relaxes blood vessels and increases blood flow, reducing heart disease. In addition, garlic boosts the immune system, prevents athlete's foot (fungus on the feet), hair loss *(with its ancillian properties),* clears acne from the skin, helps reduce weight, helps heal cold sores, inflammation, food poisoning (like E. coli and Salmonella) and hypertension and cancers.

Green Onions– Green Onions help boost your nutrition and are rich in vitamins, minerals and phytochemicals, helping with your overall bone health (Vitamins K and C; which are crucial for the growth, development and maintenance of strong bones to reduce bone fractures as well as osteoporosis), eye health (Vitamin A), immune health (DNA and cellular tissues) and heart health (Vitamin C) to reduce risk of heart disease.

Weight Loss Tip: Drink 4-5 bottles of cold water today.

BELL PEPPER

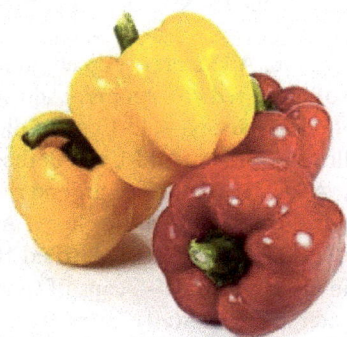

Photo Credit: posterize
FREEDIGITALPHOTOS.NET

WEEK 1, DAY 3
(CABBAGE & BARLEY SOUP)

Day 3 of Week 1: Typically makes 4-6 servings and lasts a few days, but utilize a "Small" Boiler Pot or "Small Sized Crock-Pot" (for best results) for smaller portions to watch your weight, prevent over-eating and watch your sodium (salt) intake.

Main Ingredients:
Into a Small Boiler Pot
Add a cabbage halved and 1-2 cups of organic barley

Add 1 cup of diced onion, Add 1 cup of diced green bell pepper, Add 1 cup of diced red bell pepper, Add 1 cup of corn, Add 1 cup of diced parsley, Add 1 cup of diced roma tomatoes (both yellow and red), Add 1 cup of diced celery, Add a dash of salt, Add 1/2 teaspoon of ground red pepper, Add a dash of pepper, Add 1 diced garlic clove, Add 1/2 teaspoon of thyme, Add 2 teaspoons of certified 100% organic extra-virgin olive oil, Add 4-5 cups of (purified) water (regular cold tap water is fine as well), Bring to a boil

Cook for a few hours
Cook until thoroughly heated and boiled
Serve immediately, after cooling (5-10 minutes)

Additional Notes: if desired:
Add 1 cup of any (diced) 100% certified organic, farm raised, grass fed "baked" lemon-pepper and Greek seasoned meat

Weight Loss Tip: Drink 4-5 bottles of cold water today.

PEARS

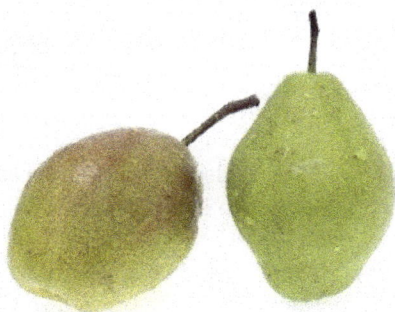

Photo Credit: phasinphoto
FREEDIGITALPHOTOS.NET

WEEK1, DAY 4
(QUINOA SALAD WITH PEARS)

Day 4 of Week 1: Almonds, Extra-Virgin Olive Oil, Chopped Parsley, Quinoa, Pears

Add 1 cup of a diced almonds into a large salad bowl, Add 2 cups of diced pears, Add 1 cup of chopped parsley, Add 1 cup of rinsed and cooked quinoa, Add 2 tablespoons of extra-virgin olive oil, Mix salad with large serving spoon until evenly mixed, Place on a bed of baby arugula on a dinner plate or in a to go container, Serve immediately

Health Notes:

Almonds – Almonds are an interesting nut. They help reduce heart attack risk, lower blood sugar, bad cholesterol, build strong bones and teeth due to their Phosphorus content, protect artery walls from damage (with their Flavonoids and Vitamin E), nourish the nervous system and the healthy fats in almonds also aid in weight loss. They also prevent certain cancers, inflammation and are known to improve skin condition.

Quinoa– Quinoa (gluten free and low in calories) is a seed that comes from a vegetable related to spinach and beets and is high in protein and even has more protein compared to some rice and wheat. Quinoa also helps promote healthy skin, energy metabolism in the brain and muscle cells, also aiding in weight loss and weight management due to its low glycemic index. It also needs washing before cooking or eating.

Arugula – Arugula is rich in Vitamins A, C and K and promotes cellular reproduction, eye health, immunity boosting, helping poor vision, improves respiratory and skin health, cleanses and detoxifies the body, helps clean out the colon and helps with bowel movements, fights cancers, boosts oxygen levels, body repair (building tissue), prevents blood clots and protects against birth defects.

Weight Loss Tip: Drink 4-5 bottles of cold water today.

TOMATOES

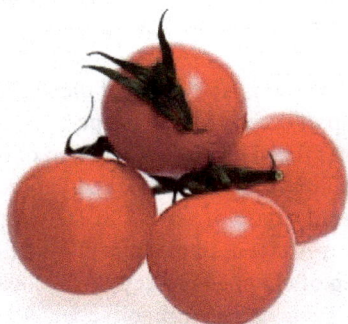

Photo Credit: Pixomar
FREEDIGITALPHOTOS.NET

WEEK 1, DAY 5
(TOMATO BASIL SOUP)

Day 5 of Week 1: Typically makes 4-6 servings and lasts a few days, but utilize a "Small" Boiler Pot or "Small Sized Crock-Pot" (for best results) for smaller portions to watch your weight, prevent over-eating and watch your sodium (salt) intake.

Main Ingredients:
Into a Small Boiler Pot
Add 4-6 diced (into small squares) large organic tomatoes and 2-3 tablespoons of organic basil

Add 1 cup of diced onion, Add 1 cup of diced green bell pepper, Add 1 cup of diced red bell pepper, Add 1 cup of corn, Add 1 cup of diced parsley, Add 1 cup of diced roma tomatoes (both yellow and red), Smoked Paprika, Add 1 cup of diced celery, Add a dash of salt, Add 1/2 teaspoon of ground red pepper, Add a dash of pepper, Add 1 diced garlic clove, Add ½ cup of chopped parsley, Add 2 teaspoons of certified 100% organic extra-virgin olive oil, Add 4-5 cups of (purified) water (regular cold tap water is fine as well), Bring to a boil

Cook for a few hours
Cook until thoroughly heated and boiled
Serve immediately, after cooling (5-10 minutes)

Additional Notes: if desired:
Add 1 cup of any (diced) 100% certified organic, farm raised, grass fed "baked" lemon-pepper and Greek seasoned meat

Weight Loss Tip: Drink 4-5 bottles of cold water today.

WALNUTS

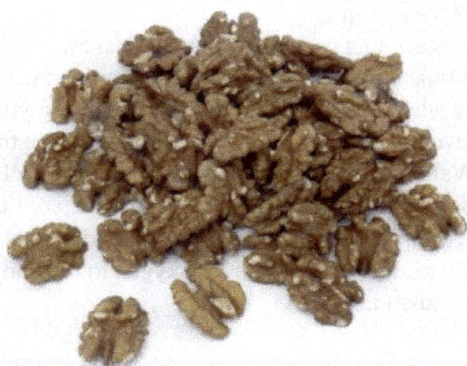

Photo Credit: Suat Eman
FREEDITIALPHOTOS.NET

Day 6 of Week 1: Walnuts, Avocado, Cilantro, Grilled Chicken Strips, Fresh Dill

Add 1 cup of a walnuts into a large salad bowl, Add 1 whole diced avocado, Add 1/2 cup of cilantro, Add 1 cup of fresh dill, Add 2-3 chopped grilled chicken strips, Mix salad with large serving spoon until evenly mixed, Place on a bed of baby arugula on a dinner plate or in a to go container, Serve immediately

Health Notes:

Walnuts – Raw nuts such as Almonds, Cashews and Walnuts have been linked to lower cholesterol, are a great snack (especially when mixed together), aid in bettering your overall health, preventing cancer risk and lowering and controlling weight. Walnuts also help protect the body from cell damage that contributes to heart disease, inflammation, are rich in Vitamin E (helping lower bad cholesterol and weight gain) and are rich in Zinc to help deliver oxygen to the body's cells and prevent anemia.

Cilantro– Most people use Cilantro (similar to "dill") in wraps, salads, pastas, pesto, guacamole and even soups. However, really, it can be used in anything. Cilantro is rich in Magnesium, Iron and antioxidants, helping the body fight aging, chronic diseases and food poisoning *(Salmonella; bacteria)*. Due to Cilantros anti-microbial properties and phytonutrients it also helps aid in curing yeast infections, kidney stones and sleep disorders.

Weight Loss Tip: Drink 4-5 bottles of cold water today.

RADISHES

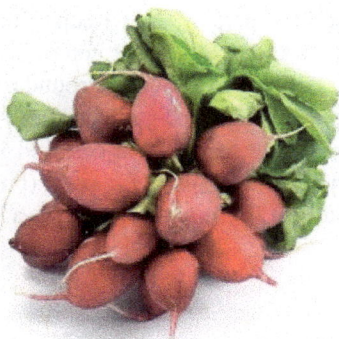

Photo Credit: Mister GC
FREEDIGITALPHOTOS.NET

WEEK 1, DAY 7
(RADISHES & GREEN-ONION SOUP)

Day 7 of Week 1: Typically makes 4-6 servings and lasts a few days, but utilize a "Small" Boiler Pot or "Small Sized Crock-Pot" (for best results) for smaller portions to watch your weight, prevent over-eating and watch your sodium (salt) intake.

Main Ingredients:
Into a Small Boiler Pot
Add 4-6 diced (into small squares) radishes and 2-3 cups of finely diced green onion or scallions

Add 1 cup of diced onion, Add 1 cup of diced green bell pepper, Add 1 cup of diced red bell pepper, Add 1 cup of corn, Add 1 cup of diced parsley, Add 1 cup of diced roma tomatoes (both yellow and red), Add 1 cup of diced celery, Add a dash of salt, Add 1/2 teaspoon of ground red pepper, Add a dash of pepper, Add 1 diced garlic clove, Add 1/2 teaspoon of thyme, Add 2 teaspoons of certified 100% organic extra-virgin olive oil, Add 4-5 cups of (purified) water (regular cold tap water is fine as well), Bring to a boil

Cook for a few hours
Cook until thoroughly heated and boiled
Serve immediately, after cooling (5-10 minutes)

Additional Notes: if desired:
Add 1 cup of any (diced) 100% certified organic, farm raised, grass fed "baked" lemon-pepper and Greek seasoned meat

Weight Loss Tip: Drink 4-5 bottles of cold water today.

WEEK 2
MIXED ROMAINE & RED
CABBAGE WEEK

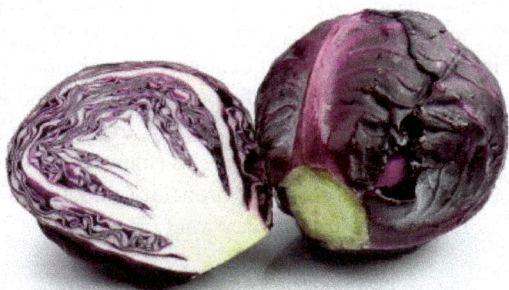

Photo Credit: SOMMAI
FREEDIGITALPHOTOS.NET

Day 1 of Week 2: **Pineapple, Green Bell Pepper, Salt/Pepper, Lemon Juice, Dill**

Add 1 cup of a diced pineapple into a large salad bowl, Add 1 cup of chopped green bell pepper, Add a dash of salt and pepper to season, Add 1/2 of a squeezed lemons juice, Add 1 cup of freshly chopped dill, Mix salad with large serving spoon until evenly mixed, Place on a bed of mixed romaine with 1/2 cup of a chopped red cabbage mixed in on a dinner plate or in a to go container, Serve immediately

Health Notes:

Dill– Dill contains anti-oxidant disease preventing properties and are rich in Vitamins A, C, Potassium, Copper, B2 (Riboflavin) as well as Zinc and beta-carotene. Dill helps with insomnia, bone health, hiccups, digestion, diarrhea and with removing excess water, gas, salt and toxins from the body. Dill also helps regulate menstrual cycles (menstrual cramps); prevents genital ulcers, infections, bronchitis and even fevers, liver and gallbladder issues (urinary tract infections).

Romaine– Rich in Omega 3's, Iron, Vitamin C (more than oranges have), Water as well as Calcium and protein, this plant also has a great source of Vitamin K. Romaine is good for your bones, teeth, eye health, night vision, impaired color vision and fighting allergies.

Red Cabbage – Red Cabbage is low in calories and fat and high in fiber and Vitamin K, making it ideal for weight loss, mental function and concentration. It also helps detoxify the body (helping to preventing arthritis, rheumatism, gout and even skin diseases), lower blood pressure and even blood sugar. Its Vitamin C content protects cells from damage and strengthen the body's muscles and tissues.

Weight Loss Tip: Drink 4-5 bottles of cold water today.

CELERY

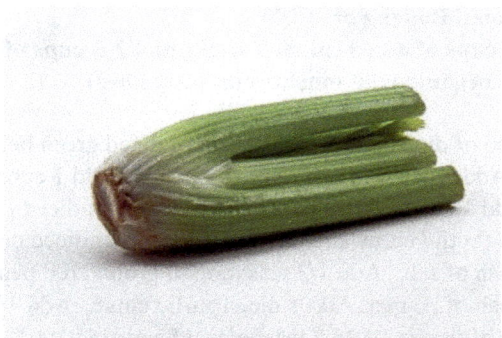

Photo Credit: James Baker
FREEDITIALPHOTOS.NET

WEEK 2, DAY 9
(SPINACH & WILD MUSHROOMS SOUP)

Day 2 of Week 2: Typically makes 4-6 servings and lasts a few days, but utilize a "Small" Boiler Pot or "Small Sized Crock-Pot" (for best results) for smaller portions to watch your weight, prevent over-eating and watch your sodium (salt) intake.

Main Ingredients:
Into a Small Boiler Pot
Add 3-4 cups of diced spinach stalks and 2-3 cups of chopped organic wild mushrooms (any kind)

Add 1 cup of diced onion, Add 1 cup of diced green bell pepper, Add 1 cup of diced red bell pepper, Add 1 cup of corn, Add 1 cup of diced parsley, Add 1 cup of diced roma tomatoes (both yellow and red), Add 1 cup of diced celery, Add a dash of salt, Add 1/2 teaspoon of ground red pepper, Add a dash of pepper, Add 1 diced garlic clove, Add 1/2 teaspoon of thyme, Add 2 teaspoons of certified 100% organic extra-virgin olive oil, Add 4-5 cups of (purified) water (regular cold tap water is fine as well), Bring to a boil

Cook for a few hours
Cook until thoroughly heated and boiled
Serve immediately, after cooling (5-10 minutes)

Additional Notes: if desired:
Add 1 cup of any (diced) 100% certified organic, farm raised, grass fed "baked" lemon-pepper and Greek seasoned meat

Weight Loss Tip: Drink 4-5 bottles of cold water today.

APPLES

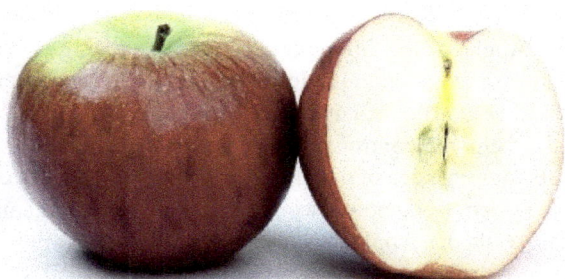

Photo Credit: Paul
FREEDIGITALPHOTOS.NET

WEEK 2, DAY 10
(SALMON CARROT LIME SALAD)

Day 3 of Week 2: Apple, Carrot, Lime Salmon, Fresh Thyme, Salt/Pepper

Add 2 diced green apples into a large salad bowl, Add 1 diced carrot, Add 1 chopped (already prepared baked piece of salmon with a limes juice cooked in), Add fresh thyme, season with a dash of salt and pepper, Mix salad with large serving spoon until evenly mixed, Place on a bed of mixed romaine with 1/2 cup of a chopped red cabbage mixed in on a dinner plate or in a to go container, Serve immediately

Health Notes:

Apples– Apples help whiten your teeth by producing saliva, assisting with reducing tooth decay, protects against cancers, gallstones, hemorrhoids, constipation and high cholesterol. They also help you control your weight, prevent cataracts, decrease your chances of developing diabetes and boost your immune system (red apples; which have an antioxidant called quercetin in them). Apples are also packed with Vitamins C, A and Flavonoids, Phosphorus, Iron and Calcium as well as Potassium to help promote heart health.

Limes – Limes are rich in Vitamin C and folate. Interestingly, you may think, the juice, fruit and peel of a lime are used to make medicines and help cure severe diarrhea. Limes also kill germs in the skin, aiding in skin care *(preventing aging);* they ease constipation and help prevent fever, urinary tract and bladder infections, ulcers, heart disease *(lowering bad cholesterol)* and even arthritis.

Thyme – Thyme helps cure colds (with its antiseptic and antibiotic properties) and improves vision because of its rich Vitamin A content and antioxidant properties promoting healthy vision.

Weight Loss Tip: Drink 4-5 bottles of cold water today.

PARSLEY

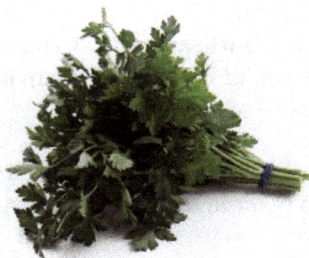

Photo Credit: James Barker
FREEDITIGALPHOTOS.NET

Day 4 of Week 2: Typically makes 4-6 servings and lasts a few days, but utilize a "Small" Boiler Pot or "Small Sized Crock-Pot" (for best results) for smaller portions to watch your weight, prevent over-eating and watch your sodium (salt) intake.

Main Ingredients:
Into a Small Boiler Pot
Add 3-4 cups of whole wheat lentils, 1 cup of roasted pumpkin seeds, 1 cup of bulgur and 1 cup of whole wheat barley, 2 tablespoons of capers

Add 1 cup of diced onion, Add 1 cup of diced green bell pepper, Add 1 cup of diced red bell pepper, Add 1 cup of corn, Add 1 cup of diced parsley, Add 1 cup of diced roma tomatoes (both yellow and red), Add 1 cup of diced cilantro, Add a dash of salt, Add 1/2 teaspoon of ground red pepper, Add a dash of pepper, Add 1 diced garlic clove, Add 1/2 teaspoon of thyme, Add 2 teaspoons of certified 100% organic extra-virgin olive oil, Add 4-5 cups of (purified) water (regular cold tap water is fine as well), Bring to a boil

Cook for a few hours
Cook until thoroughly heated and boiled
Serve immediately, after cooling (5-10 minutes)

Additional Notes: if desired:
Add 1 cup of any (diced) 100% certified organic, farm raised, grass fed "baked" lemon-pepper and Greek seasoned meat

Weight Loss Tip: Drink 4-5 bottles of cold water today.

ASPARAGUS

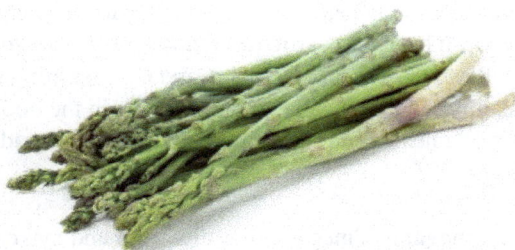

Photo Credit: SOMMAI
FREEDIGITALPHOTOS.NET

WEEK 2, DAY 12
(QUINOA PESTO SALAD)

Day 5 of Week 2: Quinoa, Pesto, Balsamic Vinegar, Roma Tomatoes, Asparagus

Add 1/2 cup of rinsed and cooked quinoa into a salad bowl, Add 2 teaspoons of pesto, Add 1 tablespoon of Balsamic Vinegar, Add 1 cup of diced roma tomatoes, Add 2-3 diced stalks of asparagus, Mix salad with large serving spoon until evenly mixed, Place on a bed of mixed romaine with 1/2 cup of a chopped red cabbage mixed in on a dinner plate or in a to go container, Serve immediately

Health Notes:

Pesto – Pesto sauce is made from olive oil, parmesan cheese, pine nuts, fresh basil and garlic *(all put into a blender to make a sauce)*. Pesto is rich in Vitamins A and C, promoting strong bones, healthy red blood cells, building tissue in the body, supporting eye health and fights disease causing free radicals in the body.

Balsamic Vinegar – Vinegar slows digestion and makes you feel fuller sooner, preventing overeating leading to weight gain and severe obesity. Balsamic Vinegar is also naturally sweetened, decreasing the need for sugar and/or additional sugar in your food or drinks. Balsamic Vinegar is also rich in antioxidants aiding in reducing cholesterol. It also helps reduce unhealthy fats and sodium in the body.

Asparagus – Asparagus contains detoxifying properties, Vitamins K, B (to help regulate blood sugar levels) A (for better vision), C, E, Iron and Inulin (a prebiotic that supports the "good" bacteria in our guts). Asparagus is also rich in fiber, low in starch and helps lower high blood pressure and heart related issues.

Weight Loss Tip: Drink 4-5 bottles of cold water today.

GARLIC

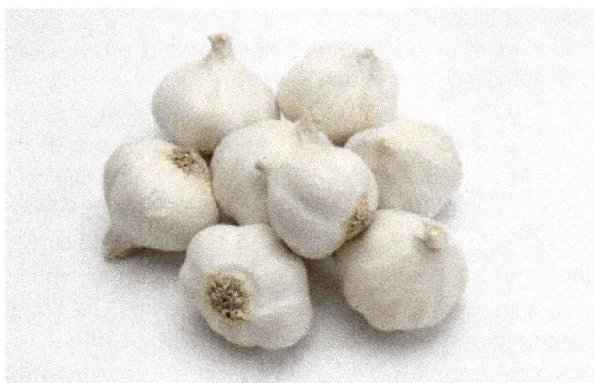

Photo Credit: Suat Eman
FREEDIGITALPHOTOS.NET

WEEK 2, DAY 13
(WHITE BEAN & ROSEMARY SOUP)

Day 6 of Week 2: Typically makes 4-6 servings and lasts a few days, but utilize a "Small" Boiler Pot or "Small Sized Crock-Pot" (for best results) for smaller portions to watch your weight, prevent over-eating and watch your sodium (salt) intake.

Main Ingredients:
Into a Small Boiler Pot
Add 3-4 cans of organic white beans and 2-3 tablespoons of finely diced rosemary

Add 1 cup of diced onion, Add 1 cup of diced green bell pepper, Add 1 cup of diced red bell pepper, Add 1 cup of corn, Add 1 cup of diced parsley, Add 1 cup of diced roma tomatoes (both yellow and red), Add 1 cup of diced celery, Add a dash of salt, Add 1/2 teaspoon of ground red pepper, Add a dash of pepper, Add 1 diced garlic clove, Add 1/2 teaspoon of thyme, Add 2 teaspoons of certified 100% organic extra-virgin olive oil, Add 4-5 cups of (purified) water (regular cold tap water is fine as well), Bring to a boil

Cook for a few hours
Cook until thoroughly heated and boiled
Serve immediately, after cooling (5-10 minutes)

Additional Notes: **if desired:**
Add 1 cup of any (diced) 100% certified organic, farm raised, grass fed "baked" lemon-pepper and Greek seasoned meat

Weight Loss Tip: Drink 4-5 bottles of cold water today.

KIWI

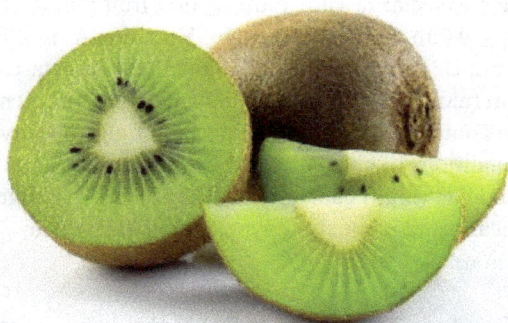

Photo Credit: SOMMAI
FREEDIGITALPHOTOS.NET

Day 7 of Week 2: Kiwi, Pineapple, Nectarines, Walnuts, Honey

Add 1 cup of a diced kiwi into a salad bowl, Add 1 cup of diced pineapple, Add 1/2 cup of diced nectarines, Add 1 cup of walnuts, Add 2 tablespoons of Honey, Mix salad with large serving spoon until evenly mixed, Place on a bed of mixed romaine with 1/2 cup of a chopped red cabbage mixed in on a dinner plate or in a to go container, Serve immediately

Health Notes:

Nectarines – Nectarines are a low calorie fruit rich in dietary fiber, Magnesium, Folate, Potassium, Vitamins A, E, C, B6, B4 (Niacin), B2 (Riboflavin), B1 (Thiamine), K, beta-carotene and Luetin (aiding in eye health), to name a few (nutrients). They also contain Chlorogenic acid which fights obesity related conditions like diabetes and cardiac issues; heart disease and bad (high) cholesterol. They also aid in digestion, cellular health and preventing hypokalemia (muscular degeneration).

Kiwi – Kiwi fruit is a small powerhouse that helps manage blood pressure because of its high level of potassium and helps with digestion. Kiwi is high in fiber and low glycemic index for weight loss, rich in immunity booster Vitamin C and carries Vitamin E for clearer skin; also fighting heart disease and cleaning toxins from the body.

Walnuts – Walnuts are an antioxidant that has an anti-inflammatory benefit which aids in preventing cardiovascular problems, cancers, type 2 diabetes (a chronic disease where there are high levels of glucose/sugar in the blood) as well as metabolic syndrome (a cluster of biochemical and physiological abnormalities that are related to type 2 diabetes).

Weight Loss Tip: Drink 4-5 bottles of cold water today.

WEEK 3
SPINACH WEEK

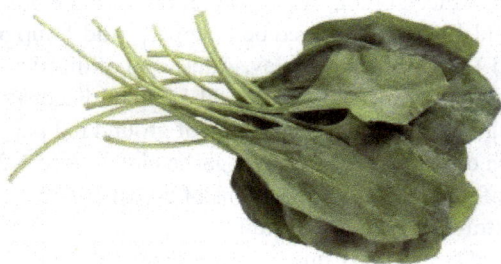

Photo Credit: Smarnd
FREEDIGITALPHOTOS.NET

Day 1 of Week 3: Typically makes 4-6 servings and lasts a few days, but utilize a "Small" Boiler Pot or "Small Sized Crock-Pot" (for best results) for smaller portions to watch your weight, prevent over-eating and watch your sodium (salt) intake.

Main Ingredients:
Into a Small Boiler Pot
Add 3-4 diced (into small squares) organic beats and 3-4 diced stalks of organic celery

Add 1 cup of diced onion, Add 1 cup of diced green bell pepper, Add 1 cup of diced red bell pepper, Add 1 cup of corn, Add 1 cup of diced parsley, Add 1 cup of diced roma tomatoes (both yellow and red), Add 1 cup of diced celery, Add a dash of salt, Add 1/2 teaspoon of ground red pepper, Add a dash of pepper, Add 1 diced garlic clove, Add 1/2 teaspoon of thyme, Add 2 teaspoons of certified 100% organic extra-virgin olive oil, Add 4-5 cups of (purified) water (regular cold tap water is fine as well), Bring to a boil

Cook for a few hours
Cook until thoroughly heated and boiled
Serve immediately, after cooling (5-10 minutes)

Additional Notes: if desired:
Add 1 cup of any (diced) 100% certified organic, farm raised, grass fed "baked" lemon-pepper and Greek seasoned meat

Weight Loss Tip: Drink 4-5 bottles of cold water today.

LIMES

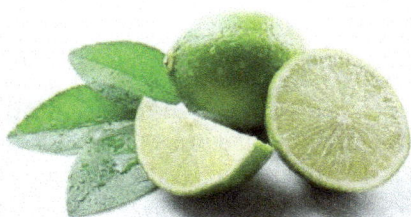

Photo Credit: Master Isolated Images
FREEDITIALPHOTOS.NET

WEEK 3, DAY 16
(TALAPIA FAJITA SALAD)

Day 2 of Week 3: Tilapia, Bowtie, Ginger, Lime, Dried Oregano

Add 1 cup of cooked (whole grain wheat) bowtie pasta into a salad bowl, Add 2 whole baked and diced tilapia, Add 1 knob of fresh ginger (small portion), Add the zest of 1 lime and the limes juice, Add 1 teaspoon of dried oregano, Mix salad with large serving spoon until evenly mixed, Place on a bed of spinach on a dinner plate or in a to go container, Serve immediately

Health Notes:

Lime – Limes are rich in Vitamin C and folate. Interestingly, you may think, the juice, fruit and peel of a lime are used to make medicines and help cure severe diarrhea. Limes also kill germs in the skin, aiding in skin care *(preventing aging);* they ease constipation and help prevent fever, urinary tract and bladder infections, ulcers, heart disease *(lowering bad cholesterol)* and even arthritis.

Oregano – Oregano is rich in Vitamins K & E, Iron, minerals, Fiber and Omega-3 fatty acids which all help in promoting overall body health, fighting acne, dandruff and even bone issues (helping to maintain bone density and preventing blood clots). Oregano also includes antioxidants to help fight infections.

Weight Loss Tip: Drink 4-5 bottles of cold water today.

ONIONS

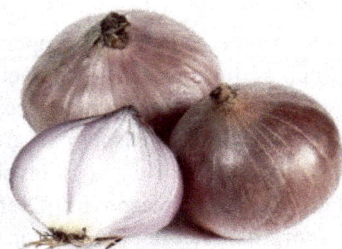

Photo Credit: HappyKanppy
FREEDIGITALPHOTOS.NET

WEEK 3, DAY 17
(SUNDRIED TOMATO & AVOCADO SOUP)

Day 3 of Week 3: Typically makes 4-6 servings and lasts a few days, but utilize a "Small" Boiler Pot or "Small Sized Crock-Pot" (for best results) for smaller portions to watch your weight, prevent over-eating and watch your sodium (salt) intake.

Main Ingredients:
Into a Small Boiler Pot
Add 6-8 cups of sun-dried tomatoes and 2-3 finely diced avocados (add in towards the end)

Add 1 cup of diced onion, Add 1 cup of diced green bell pepper, Add 1 cup of diced red bell pepper, Add 1 cup of corn, Add 1 cup of diced parsley, Add 1 cup of diced roma tomatoes (both yellow and red), Add 1 cup of diced celery, Add a dash of salt, Add 1/2 teaspoon of ground red pepper, Add a dash of pepper, Add 1 diced garlic clove, Add 1/2 teaspoon of thyme, Add 2 teaspoons of certified 100% organic extra-virgin olive oil, Add 4-5 cups of (purified) water (regular cold tap water is fine as well), Bring to a boil

Cook for a few hours
Cook until thoroughly heated and boiled
Serve immediately, after cooling (5-10 minutes)

Additional Notes: if desired:
Add 1 cup of any (diced) 100% certified organic, farm raised, grass fed "baked" lemon-pepper and Greek seasoned meat

Weight Loss Tip: Drink 4-5 bottles of cold water today.

CUCUMBERS

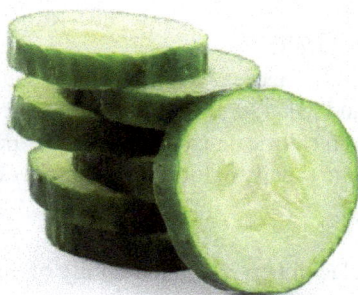

WEEK 3, DAY 18
(CUCUMBER FETA SALAD WITH BALSAMIC)
Day 4 of Week 3: Cherry Tomatoes, Black Olives, Feta Cheese, Cucumbers, Balsamic Vinegar

Add 1 cup of a diced cherry tomatoes into a salad bowl, Add 1 cup of diced black olives, Add an ounce of feta cheese, Add 1 cup of a diced cucumber, Add 1 tablespoon of balsamic vinegar to season, Mix salad with large serving spoon until evenly mixed with (whole grain wheat) bowtie pasta, Place on a dinner plate or in a to go container, Serve immediately (can also be served cold, the next day)

Health Notes:

Feta Cheese – Feta cheese is a cheese that is made with sheep or goat's milk and has a semi-hard texture. Feta cheese is rich protein and low in calories, making it ideal for pastas and salads, aiding in low daily calorie intake and **weight management.**

Cucumbers – Cucumbers are in the family of melons, squash and pumpkins. They are a great source of Vitamins K, C, A and B and are made up 95% water and are great for the eyes, skin and hair due to their anti-inflammatory properties and hair growth stimulation. They also help fight cancers (ovarian, uterine, breast as well as prostate) and aid in **weight loss**, digestion, blood pressure control, cholesterol reduction and joint pain relief (that is associated with arthritis). Cucumbers also dissolve kidney stones and rid the body of waste products.

Goat Cheese – Goat cheese is rich in Calcium, Vitamins A & K, Thiamin, Niacin and even Phosphorus. Fats found in goat milk are easier for the body to process than cow's milk, promoting an overall healthy diet (body).

Weight Loss Tip: Drink 4-5 bottles of cold water today.

CORN

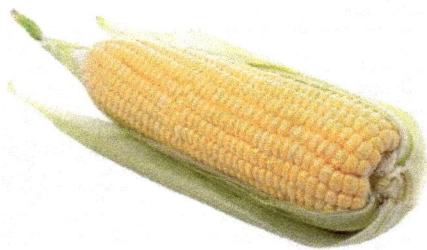

Photo Credit: SOMMAI
FREEDIGITALPHOTOS.NET

Day 5 of Week 3: Typically makes 4-6 servings and lasts a few days, but utilize a "Small" Boiler Pot or "Small Sized Crock-Pot" (for best results) for smaller portions to watch your weight, prevent over-eating and watch your sodium (salt) intake.

Main Ingredients:
Into a Small Boiler Pot
Add 3-4 cups diced asparagus stalks

Add 1 cup of diced onion, Add 1 cup of diced green bell pepper, Add 1 cup of diced red bell pepper, Add 1 cup of corn, Add 1 cup of diced parsley, Add 1 cup of diced roma tomatoes (both yellow and red), Add 1 cup of diced celery, Add a dash of salt, Add 1/2 teaspoon of ground red pepper, Add a dash of pepper, Add 1 diced garlic clove, Add 1/2 teaspoon of thyme, Add 2 teaspoons of certified 100% organic extra-virgin olive oil, Add 4-5 cups of (purified) water (regular cold tap water is fine as well), Bring to a boil

Cook for a few hours
Cook until thoroughly heated and boiled
Serve immediately, after cooling (5-10 minutes)

Additional Notes: if desired:
Add 1 cup of any (diced) 100% certified organic, farm raised, grass fed "baked" lemon-pepper and Greek seasoned meat

Weight Loss Tip: Drink 4-5 bottles of cold water today.

AVOCADOS

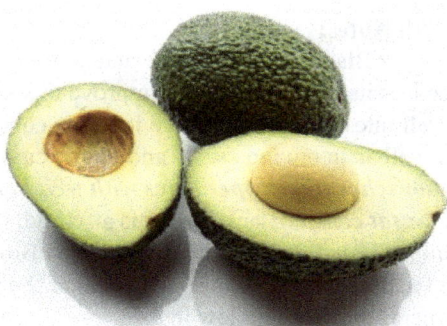

Photo Credit: MASTER ISOLATED IMAGES
FREEDIGITALPHOTOS.NET

WEEK 3, DAY 20
(SHRIMP AVOCADO SALAD)

Day 6 of Week 3: Black Pepper, Avocado, Shrimp, Cilantro, Sesame Oil

Add 1 cup of a whole diced avocado into a salad bowl, Add 1/2 cup of cilantro, Add 2 tablespoons of sesame oil, Add a dash of black pepper and sea salt to season, Add 2 cups of diced (cooked; baked or sautéed in butter) shrimp (tail removed) Mix salad with large serving spoon until evenly mixed, Place on a bed of spinach on a dinner plate or in a to go container, Serve immediately

Health Notes:

(Black) Pepper – Black pepper (a spice and a medicine) is beneficial the less its heated and helps improve digestion and promote overall intestinal health; I love it on my cobb salads and soups as well as in my tuna salad and on my custom made egg salad *sandwiches (the pepper helps with weight loss by breaking down fat cells).* Black pepper is also high in dietary fiber, B Vitamins (B1, B2, B3, B6, B12 and even Biotin (for hair, skin and nail health) & Folate), A Vitamins D and E, including mineral proteins and low in calories. This pepper also comes in white. Black pepper helps with relief from respiratory disorder, coughs, indigestion, anemia, dental diseases, constipation and even diarrhea.

Sesame Oil - Sesame seeds contain B Vitamins, Calcium, Iron, Manganese, Copper, Magnesium, Fiber, Zinc, Vitamins B6, Protein, Phosphorous as well as Thiamin. The Vitamins and Minerals in Sesame Seeds / Sesame Seed Oil is great for oral health (reducing the amount of streptococcus mutants in teeth plaque and mouth saliva), preventing diabetes, reducing blood pressure, preventing DNA damage and cancers. They also detoxify the body and prevent iron deficiency.

Weight Loss Tip: Drink 4-5 bottles of cold water today.

BROCCOLI

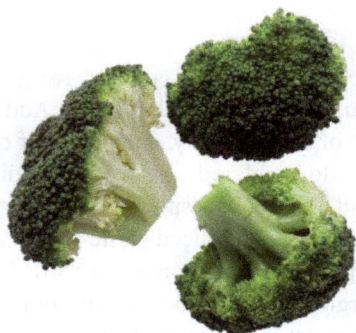

Photo Credit: phasinphoto
FREEDIGITALPHOTOS.NET

WEEK 3, DAY 21
(BROCCOLI SOUP)

Day 7 of Week 3: Typically makes 4-6 servings and lasts a few days, but utilize a "Small" Boiler Pot or "Small Sized Crock-Pot" (for best results) for smaller portions to watch your weight, prevent over-eating and watch your sodium (salt) intake.

Main Ingredients:
Into a Small Boiler Pot
Add one full pot of organic (washed & rinsed) broccoli (cut into florets)

Add 1 cup of diced onion, Add 1 cup of diced green bell pepper, Add 1 cup of diced red bell pepper, Add 1 cup of corn, Add 1 cup of diced parsley, Add 1 cup of diced roma tomatoes (both yellow and red), Add 1 cup of diced celery, Add a dash of salt, Add 1/2 teaspoon of ground red pepper, Add a dash of pepper, Add 1 diced garlic clove, Add 1/2 teaspoon of thyme, Add 2 teaspoons of certified 100% organic extra-virgin olive oil, Add 4-5 cups of (purified) water (regular cold tap water is fine as well), Bring to a boil

Cook for a few hours
Cook until thoroughly heated and boiled
Serve immediately, after cooling (5-10 minutes)

Additional Notes: if desired:
Add 1 cup of any (diced) 100% certified organic, farm raised, grass fed "baked" lemon-pepper and Greek seasoned meat

Weight Loss Tip: Drink 4-5 bottles of cold water today.

CONGRATULATIONS ON YOUR NEW YOU!

*Keep up the great work by continuing
on with my two newest books, "The 21 Day Smoothie Fast"
and the "The 7 Day Detox"*

INDEX OF RECIPES

DAY 1	42	DAY 12	64
DAY 2	44	DAY 13	66
DAY 3	46	DAY 14	68
DAY 4	48	DAY 15	70
DAY 5	50	DAY 16	72
DAY 6	52	DAY 17	74
DAY 7	54	DAY 18	76
DAY 8	56	DAY 19	78
DAY 9	58	DAY 20	80
DAY 10	60	DAY 21	82
DAY 11	62		